DIAGNOSIS AND TREATMENT OF PARKINSON'S DISEASE.

By

DR DOUGLAS JASON

Before this document is duplicated or reproduced in any manner, the publisher's consent must be gained.

Therefore, the contents within can neither be stored electronically, transferred, nor kept in a database. Neither in part nor in full can the document be copied, scanned, faxed, or retained without approval from the publisher or creator.

TABLE OF CONTENTS

ABOUT THE AUTHOR

INTRODUCTION

TABLE OF CONTENTS

DIAGNOSIS AND TREATMENT OF PARKINSON'S DISEASE.

INTRODUCTION

Part 1:Diagnosis Of Parkinson's Illness.

Part 2:Treatment AND Drugs.

Part 3: Way of life and home cures.

Part 4: Alternative medication.

Part 5: Adapting and support.

Part 6: Planning for your arrangement.

CONCLUSION.

ABOUT THE AUTHOR

Dr. DOUGLAS JASON is a certified dietician who has a strong passion for wellness and a big eagerness to help people all over the world. He uses healthy food, herbs, sauce, and other useful tools to help mankind realize its overall goal of optimum health.

INTRODUCTION

Parkinson's sickness, a neurodegenerative problem, presents an impressive test in the domain of clinical science. As how we might interpret its complexities develops, so does the significance of precise findings and compelling treatment. This paper digs into the complex scene of Parkinson's illness, investigating the subtleties of its findings and the developing scene of helpful intercessions.

Part 1:Diagnosis Of Parkinson's Illness.

As of now, there is no particular test to analyze Parkinson's sickness. A finding is made by a specialist prepared in sensory system conditions, known as a nervous system specialist. A conclusion of Parkinson's depends on your clinical history, a survey of your side effects, and a neurological and actual test.

An individual from your medical care group might propose a particular single-photon emanation mechanized tomography (SPECT) filter called a dopamine carrier (DAT) check. Albeit this can assist with supporting the doubt that you have Parkinson's illness, it is your side effects and consequences of a neurological test that at last decide the right conclusion. A great many people don't need a DAT filter. Your consideration group might arrange lab tests, for example, blood tests, to preclude different circumstances that might be causing your side effects. Imaging tests like an X-ray, ultrasound of the mind, and PET sweeps might be utilized to assist with precluding different issues. Imaging tests aren't especially useful for diagnosing Parkinson's sickness.

As well as looking at you, an individual from your medical services group might give you carbidopa-levodopa (Rytary, Sinemet, others), a

Parkinson's sickness medication. You should be given an adequate portion to show the advantage, as getting low dosages for a little while isn't dependable. Huge improvement with this medication will frequently affirm your finding of Parkinson's infection.

In some cases, it requires investment to analyze Parkinson's sickness. Medical care experts might suggest ordinary subsequent meetings with nervous system specialists prepared in development issues to assess your condition and side effects over the long run and analyze Parkinson's sickness. Notwithstanding, another test might not be too far off. Scientists are concentrating on a Parkinson's test that can distinguish the illness before side effects start. The test is called an alpha-synuclein seed intensification measure. In a recent report, specialists tried the spinal liquid of more than 1,000 individuals to search for bunches of the protein alpha-synuclein. Alpha-synuclein is found in Lewy bodies. It structures bunches that the body can't separate. The clusters spread and harm synapses.

Alpha-synuclein clusters are a trademark indication of Parkinson's illness. The test precisely recognized individuals with Parkinson's illness 87.7% of the time. The test additionally was exceptionally touchy for identifying individuals in danger of Parkinson's illness. This investigation of the alpha-synuclein seed enhancement examination was the biggest up to this point. A few scientists say the review might be a unique advantage for Parkinson's sickness determination, examination, and therapy preliminaries. Be that as it may, bigger examinations are required. There's trust among scientists that later on, the test should be possible utilizing blood tests as opposed to spinal liquid.

Part 2:Treatment AND Drugs.

Parkinson's sickness can't be restored, however, drugs can assist with controlling the side effects, frequently decisively. In a few further developed cases, medical procedures might be encouraged.
Your medical care group additionally may suggest way of life changes, particularly progressing high-impact workouts. Now and again, exercise-based recuperation that spotlights extension and

extending is significant. A discourse language pathologist might assist with further developing discourse issues.

Meds

Meds might assist you with overseeing issues with strolling, development, and quake. These medications increment or substitute for dopamine.

Individuals with Parkinson's illness have low degrees of cerebrum dopamine. Be that as it may, dopamine can't be given straightforwardly because it can't enter the mind.

You might have a huge improvement in your side effects after starting Parkinson's illness treatment. After some time, in any case, the advantages of medications now and again decrease or become less predictable. You can generally still control your side effects well.

Medications your consideration group might recommend include:

Carbidopa-levodopa (Rytary, Sinemet, Duopa, others).

Levodopa, the best Parkinson's sickness medication, is a characteristic substance that passes into the cerebrum and is switched over completely to dopamine.

 Levodopa is joined with carbidopa (Lodosyn), which shields levodopa from early transformation to dopamine outside the cerebrum. This forestalls or decreases secondary effects like sickness.

Aftereffects might incorporate queasiness or dizziness when you stand, called orthostatic hypotension.

After years, as your infection advances, the advantage from levodopa might diminish, with a propensity to fluctuate, likewise called "wearing off."

Likewise, you might encounter compulsory developments known as dyskinesia in the wake of taking higher doses of levodopa. Your consideration group might reduce your portion or change the hours of your dosages to control these impacts.

Except if told in any case by your medical services group, carbidopa-levodopa is best taken while starving assuming you have progressed Parkinson's sickness.

Breathe in carbidopa-levodopa. Inbrija is a brand-name medication conveying carbidopa-levodopa in a breathed-in structure. It might assist with overseeing side effects that emerge when drugs taken by mouth unexpectedly quit working during the day. Carbidopa-levodopa imbuement. Duopa is a brand-name medication joining carbidopa and levodopa. Notwithstanding, it's controlled through taking care of a cylinder that conveys the medication in a gel structure straightforwardly to the small digestive system.

 Duopa is for patients with further developed Parkinson's

who answer carbidopa-
levodopa but who have a ton
of vacillations in their reaction.
Since Duopa is persistently
mixed, the blood levels of the
two medications stay
consistent.

 The situation of the cylinder
requires a little surgery.
Chances related to having the
cylinder incorporate the
cylinder dropping out or
diseases at the mixture site.

Dopamine agonists. Dissimilar
to levodopa, dopamine

agonists don't change into dopamine. All things being equal, they mirror dopamine impacts in the cerebrum.

Dopamine agonists aren't quite as powerful as levodopa in treating side effects. In any case, they last longer and might be utilized with levodopa to smooth the occasional now-and-again impact of levodopa.

Dopamine agonists incorporate pramipexole (Mirapex emergency room) and rotigotine (Neupro), which is given as a fix. Apomorphine (Apokyn) is a short-acting dopamine agonist shot utilized for speedy help.

 A portion of the results of dopamine agonists resemble the symptoms of carbidopa-levodopa. Be that as it may, they additionally can incorporate mind flights, lethargy, and habitual ways of behaving like hypersexuality, betting, and eating. On the off chance that you're taking these drugs and you act in a manner that is bizarre for you, converse with your medical care group.

Monoamine oxidase B (MAO B) inhibitors. These meds incorporate selegiline (Zelapar), rasagiline (Azilect), and safinamide (Xadago). They assist with forestalling the breakdown of cerebrum dopamine by repressing the mind compound monoamine oxidase B (MAO B). This catalyst separates cerebrum dopamine. Selegiline given with levodopa might assist with forestalling wearing off.

Results of MAO B inhibitors might incorporate cerebral pains, queasiness, or sleep deprivation. When added to carbidopa-levodopa, these meds increase the gamble of pipedreams.

These meds are not frequently utilized in the mix with most antidepressants or certain aggravation medications because of possibly serious yet uncommon responses. Check with your medical care group

before taking any extra drugs
with an MAO B inhibitor.

Catechol O-methyltransferase
(COMT) inhibitors.
Entacapone (Comtan) and
opicapone (Ongentys) are the
essential prescriptions from
this class. This medication
gently draws out the impact of
levodopa treatment by
impeding a catalyst that
separates dopamine.

 After Effects, including an
expanded gamble of
compulsory developments

called dyskinesia, essentially result from an upgraded levodopa impact. Opposite incidental effects incorporate looseness of the bowels, sickness, or retching.

 Tolcapone (Tasmar) is one more COMT inhibitor that is seldom recommended because of the gamble of serious liver harm and liver disappointment.

Anticholinergics. These medications were utilized for a long time to assist with controlling the quake-related to Parkinson's illness. A few anticholinergic meds are accessible, including benztropine (Cogentin) or trihexyphenidyl.

 Notwithstanding, their unobtrusive advantages are much of the time offset by aftereffects like weakened memory, disarray, fantasies, clogging, dry mouth, and disabled pee.

Amantadine. Medical care experts might recommend

amantadine (Govori) alone to give momentary help of side effects of gentle, beginning phase Parkinson's illness. It likewise might be given with carbidopa-levodopa treatment during the later phases of Parkinson's sickness to control compulsory developments called dyskinesia incited via carbidopa-levodopa.

 Secondary effects might include a change in skin tone, lower leg expansion, or mind flight.

Adenosine receptor adversaries (A2A receptor bad guys). These medications target regions in the mind that manage the dopamine reaction and permit more dopamine to be delivered. Istradefylline (Nourianz) is one of the A2A adversary drugs. Nuplazid (Pimavanserin). This medication is utilized to treat visualizations and hallucinations that can happen with Parkinson's illness. Specialists don't know how it functions.

Surgeries

Profound cerebrum feeling. In profound cerebrum feeling (DBS), specialists embed terminals into a particular piece of the mind. The terminals are associated with a generator embedded in the chest close to the collarbone. The generator sends electrical heartbeats to the mind and may diminish Parkinson's infection side effects.

 Your medical services group might change your settings as it is important to treat your condition. The medical procedure implies chances, including diseases, stroke, or cerebrum drain. Certain individuals experience issues with the DBS framework or have entanglements because of excitement. An individual from your medical care group might have to change or supplant a few pieces of the framework.

Profound cerebrum feeling is most frequently proposed to individuals with cutting-edge Parkinson's illness who have shaky reactions to levodopa.

DBS can balance out medication variances, lessen or end compulsory developments called dyskinesia, decrease quakes, diminish inflexibility, and further develop developments.

 DBS is viable for controlling changing reactions to levodopa or for controlling dyskinesia that doesn't improve with medication changes.

 Nonetheless, DBS isn't useful for issues that don't answer

levodopa treatment separated from quakes. Quakes might be constrained by DBS regardless of whether the quake is extremely receptive to levodopa.

 Even though DBS might give a supported advantage to Parkinson's side effects, it doesn't hold Parkinson's illness back from advancing.

High-level medicines X-ray-directed centred ultrasound (MRgFUS) is an insignificantly intrusive treatment that has assisted certain individuals with Parkinson's sickness to oversee quakes. Ultrasound is directed by an X-ray of the region in the cerebrum where the quakes start. The ultrasound waves are at an exceptionally high temperature and consume regions that are adding to the quakes.

Part 3: Way of life and home cures.

You'll have to work intimately with your medical care group to find a Parkinson's therapy plan that offers you the best help from side effects with the least secondary effects.

Certain medications can exacerbate your side effects, so if it's not too much trouble, examine with your consideration group any prescriptions you right now take.

A certain way of life changes likewise may assist with making living with Parkinson's sickness more straightforward.

Smart dieting

While no food or blend of food varieties has been demonstrated to help in Parkinson's sickness, a few food sources might assist with facilitating a portion of the side effects. For instance, eating food sources high in fibre and drinking a lot of liquids can assist with forestalling clogging which is normal in Parkinson's illness.

A fair eating routine likewise gives supplements, for example, omega-3 unsaturated fats, that may be useful for individuals with Parkinson's infection.

Work out

Practising may build your muscle strength, adaptability, and equilibrium. Practice can further develop your prosperity and lessen melancholy or uneasiness.

Your medical care group might propose that you work with an actual specialist to become familiar with an activity program that works for you. You likewise may attempt activities like strolling, swimming, cultivating, moving, water vigorous exercise, or extending.

Parkinson's sickness can upset your feeling of equilibrium, making it hard to stroll with your typical walk. Exercise might work on your equilibrium. These ideas additionally may help:

Do whatever it takes not to move excessively fast.

Hold back nothing to strike the floor first while you're strolling.

If you notice yourself pausing, pau pause at your stance. Standing upright is ideal.

Thoroughly search before you, not straightforwardly down, while strolling.
Staying away from falls
In the later phases of the illness, you might fall all the more without any problem. You might be rattled by only a little push or knock. The accompanying ideas might help:
Turn around as opposed to turning your body over your feet.
Disseminate your weight equally between the two feet and don't incline.

Try not to convey things while you walk.

Abstain from strolling in reverse.

Everyday living exercises
Everyday living exercises like dressing, eating, washing, and composing can be hard for individuals with Parkinson's illness. A word-related specialist can show you methods that make day-to-day existence simpler.

If you are experiencing difficulty talking, a language teacher might have the option to help. Many individuals with

Parkinson's illness have discourse hardships, for example, a sluggish, frail voice, issues with consonants, slurred discourse, a soft tone that has a droning with little articulation, and unseemly hushes. A language teacher might have the option to assist with these issues.

Part 4: Alternative medication.

Strong treatments can assist with facilitating a portion of the side effects and confusion of Parkinson's sickness, like torment, weariness, and gloom. At the point when acted in the mix with your medicines, these treatments could woo on your satisfaction
Knead. Knead treatment can diminish muscle strain and advance unwinding. This treatment, be that as it may, is

seldom covered by health care coverage.

Jujitsu. An old type of Chinese activity, jujitsu utilizes slow, streaming movements that might further develop adaptability, equilibrium, and muscle strength. Kendo likewise may assist with forestalling falls. A few types of judo are customized for individuals of all ages or states of being.

A review showed that yoga might work on the equilibrium of individuals with gentle to direct Parkinson's infection more than extending and obstruction preparation.

Yoga. In yoga, delicate extending developments and stances might expand your adaptability and equilibrium. You might adjust most postures to accommodate your actual capacities.
Alexander strategy. This strategy which centers around muscle stance, equilibrium, and contemplating how you use muscles may diminish muscle strain and agony.

Reflection. In contemplation, you unobtrusively reflect and zero in your psyche on a thought or picture. Reflection might diminish pressure and torment and work on your feeling of prosperity.

Pet treatment. Having a canine or feline might build your adaptability and development and work on your profound well-being.

Unwinding methods. These practices assist with bringing down your pulse, diminish your pulse, and further develop muscle tone.

Part 5: Adapting and support.

Living with any constant ailment can be troublesome, and it's normal to feel irate, discouraged or deterred on occasion. Parkinson's sickness can be significantly baffling as strolling, talking, and in any event, eating becomes more troublesome and tedious. Wretchedness is normal in individuals with Parkinson's sickness. Yet, upper medications can assist with facilitating the side effects of despondency, so talk with your medical services group if you're feeling perseveringly miserable or sad.

Even though loved ones can be your best partners, the comprehension of individuals who understand what you're going through can be particularly useful. Support bunches aren't a great fit for everybody. Nonetheless, for some individuals with Parkinson's sickness and their families, a care group can be a decent asset for reasonable data about Parkinson's illness. Likewise, bunches offer a spot for you to find individuals who are going through comparative circumstances and can uphold you.

Attempting to keep up with a portion of your standard exercises might be useful. Mean to do however many things as would be prudent that you could do before the beginning of Parkinson's illness. Center around the present and attempt to keep an uplifting outlook.

To find out about help bunches locally, converse with your medical care group, a Parkinson's infection social labourer, or a nearby general well-being medical caretaker. Or on the other hand contact the Parkinson's Establishment or the American Parkinson Illness Affiliation.

You and your family likewise may profit from conversing with emotional well-being proficient, for example, a clinician or social labourer prepared to work with individuals who have constant circumstances.

Part 6: Planning for your arrangement.

You're probably going to initially see a medical services proficient. You may then be referred to a specialist preferred system issues, called a nervous system specialist.

Since there's in many cases a great deal to examine, it's smart to plan for your arrangement. Here is data to assist you with preparing for your arrangement.

What you can do

Record any side effects you're encountering, including any that might appear to be inconsequential to the justification for which you booked the arrangement.

Record key individual data, including any significant burdens or ongoing life-altering events.

Make a rundown of all prescriptions, nutrients, and enhancements that you're taking.

Ask a relative or companion to accompany you, if conceivable.

Once in a while, it tends to be hard to recollect all the data given to you during an arrangement. Somebody who goes with you might recollect something that you missed or neglected.

Record inquiries to pose during your arrangement.

Your experience with your consideration group is restricted, so setting up a rundown of inquiries quite a bit early will assist you with capitalizing on your time together. For Parkinson's infection, a few fundamental inquiries to pose include:

What's the most probable reason for my side effects?

Are there other potential causes?

What sorts of tests do I want? Do these tests require any extraordinary readiness?

How does Parkinson's illness generally advance?

Will I ultimately need long-haul care?

What medicines are accessible,
and which do you suggest for me?
What kinds of secondary effects
might I at any point anticipate from
treatment?
On the off chance that the
treatment doesn't work or quits
working, do I have extra choices?
I have other ailments. How might I
best deal with these
circumstances together?
Are there any pamphlets or other
written words that I can bring back
home with me? What sites do you
suggest?
Notwithstanding the inquiries that
you've arranged to pose to your
consideration group, make sure to

questions that happen to you during your arrangement.

What's in store from your primary care physician

Your medical services group is probably going to pose a few inquiries. Being prepared to answer them might hold time to go over any focuses you need to invest more energy in. You might be inquired:

When did you initially start encountering side effects?

Do you have side effects constantly, or do they travel every which way?

Does anything appear to work on your side effects?

Does anything appear to exacerbate your side effects? doesn't support organizations or items. Publicizing income upholds our not-for-profit mission.

CONCLUSION.

All in all, the excursion of diagnosing and treating Parkinson's illness is a unique cycle set apart by progressions in innovation, pharmacology, and a developing cognizance of the hidden neurobiology. While challenges continue, the steps made as of late rouse trust for further developed results and a more promising time to come for those impacted by this complicated problem.

As we stand at the crossing
point of clinical development
and humane consideration, the
journey for additional exact
determinations and improved
treatment modalities keeps,
offering beams of confidence
for people living with
Parkinson's infection.

www.ingramcontent.com/pod-product-compliance
Lightning Source LLC
Chambersburg PA
CBHW071106260726
48661CB00006B/2487